MW00931759

The Pain

Within Me

My Battle with Fibromyalgia

By Lawawn Dunbar

Copyright© 2019 Lawawn Dunbar

Published and Printed in the United States of America

Disclaimer: This book contains information that is intended to help the readers be better informed consumers of health care. It is presented as general advice on health and body care. Always consult your doctor for your individual needs. Before beginning any new diet or exercise program it is recommended that you seek medical advice from your personal physician. This book is not intended to be a substitute for the medical advice of a licensed physician. The reader should consult with their doctor in any matters relating to his/her health.

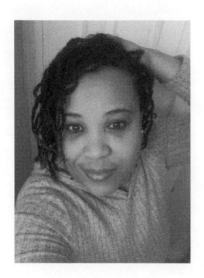

The purpose of this book is to give people the knowledge of how black American women suffer with chronic pain. Black women are often labeled with the stigma of being lazy addicts who are just looking for a fix. But this couldn't be any further from the truth. We suffer just like anyone else, and our struggles with pain are just as valid. **-Lawawn**

I want all of my family and friends who aren't already aware, to know that I have chronic pain. My days are very hard at times. I know I don't look sick, but I am. I need you all to know that I'm trying my best to stay focused and keep pushing through. I have good and bad days. So please don't get upset when I cancel things that you invite me to. it's not that I don't want to hangout it's just that I can't. I'm not looking for sympathy or anyone's pity I just need your support.

-Thank you.

The Pain Within Me

The Pain Within Me

∞

I've been dealing with symptoms of fibromyalgia (fy-bro-my-al-gia) since 2003. I was suffering with chronic pain throughout my entire body, from my lower back to my legs. The pain was excruciating but doctors were clueless as to what was wrong with me. Some recommended that I change my eating habits and that the pain was just in my head. So as the years went by the pain got worse. I still had no clue what was going on. In 2012, I went to the emergency room in what felt like the worst pain I had ever experienced. I felt like I was on fire from head to toe. Once I finally saw a doctor, they were still stumped. Still, no answers. That's when they recommended that I see a specialist. I made an appointment with a local Rheumatologist. After running several tests, he determined that I had fibromyalgia.

Fibromyalgia, also known as fibro myositis and fibrositis, is a disorder characterized by widespread musculoskeletal pain accompanied by fatigue, sleep, memory and mood issues. Researchers believe that fibromyalgia amplifies painful sensations by affecting the way your brain processes pain signals. Symptoms sometimes begin after a physical trauma, surgery, infection or significant psychological stress. In other cases, symptoms gradually accumulate over time with no single triggering event. The term fibromyalgia is from New Latin fibro-fibrous tissues, myo- muscle, algia-pain = muscle connective tissue pain. Many people experience cognitive dysfunction (fibro fog) which causes problems concentrating. There is strong evidence that major depression is associated with fibromyalgia. Neurogenic inflammation has been proposed as a contributing factor to fibromyalgia. The first clinical study of the characteristics of fibromyalgia syndrome was in 1981. In 1981 trials of medications for fibromyalgia were proposed and published. People with fibromyalgia use twice as much pain related medications as those without it. Neurologist and pain specialist tend to view fibromyalgia as a pathology due to dysfunction of muscles and connective tissue as well as functional abnormalities in the central nervous system.

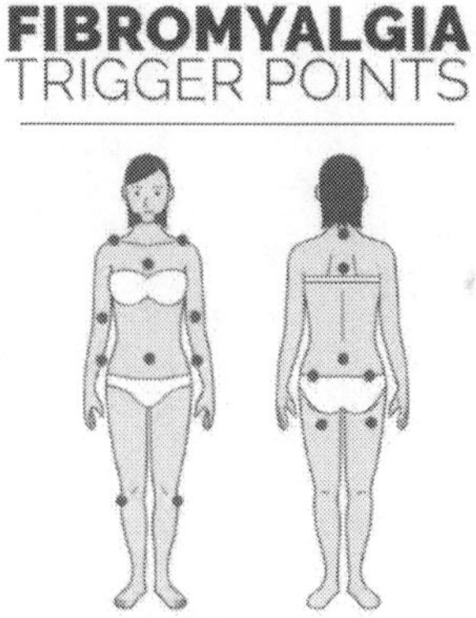

He broke everything down in detail, explaining why I had been in so much pain for so long. He also explained the cause of the burning sensations I had been experiencing. They are called “fibro flare ups”. He told me that I needed to do research on this condition that I would be living with for the rest of my life. A wave of sadness overcame me when he told me that there was no cure. The Dr. offered his apologies, and was very sympathetic about my struggles. He felt bad that I had gone so long with chronic pain and no answers. But now, I finally understood and had the answers that I longed for.

The breakouts and the burning sensation that I experience is like nothing you could ever imagine. As time went on, I had to open up to my family and tell them about my battle with fibromyalgia. Some were very sympathetic and supportive. Others, not so much. They felt that I was letting this pain ruin my life, and I couldn't understand why they felt this way. It hurt me to know that those I cared about, failed to understand what I was going through. This caused me to distance myself, and stay away from family gatherings for a while. But the pain was so bad, I couldn't go to family functions or even hangout with friends even if I wanted to. If I did decide to attending outings and family events, I would have to take my meds which made me drowsy. Once the side effects set in, I would have to excuse myself and leave. Sometimes I feel that people hesitate to invite me out because of my chronic pain. But I don't blame them. The last thing anyone wants is to ruin the fun.

Sometimes the pain is so bad, that I have to stay in bed all day. Having to be on several medications just to have a normal day is a depressing reality for me. At times, I lay in bed and cry as my struggle with this pain overwhelms me. The life I once had is gone, and simple things I used to enjoy like going to the mall, have become extremely overwhelming. When I do go to the store, I have to hold on to a shopping cart just to get through my shopping errands. People look at me and see my smile, assuming that everything is okay. But what they don't realize is that I smile to hide my pain. I smile to keep the tears from filling my eyes. I can't even take a shower without the pain ravishing me, and those who don't live in my shoes could never grasp what my life is like.

∞

I go to my doctors' appointments and it's an endless cycle of meds and more meds. Since there is no cure, pain management is my only solution. My hands swell up when I'm too active, and I can't sit nor stand for long periods of time. I sometimes wonder what I did to deserve this curse. I throw my head back and ask God "Why me?" Why must I suffer? I suffer from the moment I wake up, until I lay my head down at night and close my eyes. During the summer months, I keep my body covered due to dark spots I have because of break outs. My friends and family can often tell when I'm having a flare up, because my face will visibly swell.

This disease is awful. They make you get injections constantly and it's so much to bear. It breaks my heart that I was suffering for so long and nobody knew what was wrong with me. They would say it was my back.

Yes, it's true that I have back problems too, but that wasn't it. I get so tired of taking medication every single day. The medication keeps me drowsy and I can't work because I'm always in pain. I have to lay down and rest for most of the day. If I attempt any long-term activities the pain will plague me, and I can't take it.

I thank God that I have such a wonderful husband who is by my side every day. It really helps when you have a great support system. My lovely children, my cousin and my best friend are also my #1 support. I feel bad when I engage in these social media groups and women say they don't have anyone supporting them. We all need that support to get through it. The battle with fibromyalgia can lead to long periods of depressive episodes. Along with my depression, I also suffer from degenerative disc disease and a few other things. All which are very painful. I stay up at night, praying to God and asking him to help me through the pain. You have to find ways to keep yourself at peace with this. I would never wish this pain on anyone.

When I heard that children also struggle with fibromyalgia, it broke my heart. As an adult, I can hardly make it through the day with this disease, so it shatters my heart to even imagine a child going through this. About a year ago doctors suspected that my eight-year-old daughter had it! I cried so hard and prayed with everything in me that she wouldn't have to suffer with this. Thank God it was just a false alarm, but she will get tested every year just to be on the safe side. I was so scared for my baby. They say fibromyalgia can be hereditary, and stems from overactive nerves that cause constant pain in your body. It's mostly effects women, but men also suffer, just not in high numbers compared to us.

A testimonial from a friend of mine who also struggles with fibromyalgia:

"Being diagnosed with fibromyalgia, almost a year-and-a-half ago I got sick. It seemed as if the symptoms where coming on fairly fast and one right after the other. I had a visit to the emergency room and from there I started seeing all sorts of specialists because I had terrible head pain, fatigue, swelling, joint pain, muscle pain as well as head pressure . The swelling that I had in my legs were fluid. This wasn't a scary experience

14

because we didn't know if it was something serious. I was put on so many different meds and at one point I couldn't tell whether it was helping or not. I couldn't walk from one end of a store to the other. Couldn't handle the heat. I would become doused in sweat it would almost take my breath away and of course I was very scared. Through my testing I found out that my thyroid was hyper at the time. But a few months later of not being able to get it under control we realized that I actually had a virus. It was hyper then hypo then non-active. We were finally able to gain control of my thyroid but unfortunately the virus in my thyroid threw me into fibromyalgia. I had the same exact symptoms that one would have with lupus and even after my thyroid became normal the pain never left. Almost crippling pain. I continue to see my rheumatologist until she realized that I had fibromyalgia. I was prescribed two more prescriptions, but I haven't started. I'm a little nervous about the side effects. I'm learning how to function with this diagnosis and maybe I will at some point start the meds once I'm sure that it won't cause any other issues."

Over the years it has progressed, that's what the doctors tell me. I can see the movements in my legs and arms. The flare ups are everyday now. They give me all this medication, but it does nothing but put me to sleep. I've been considering all natural alternatives. I'm desperate for relief. I'm tired of my body feeling like it's on fire and the fatigue is terrible. Most nights I might get about 3-4 hours of sleep. If I do get 8 hours, I'll usually still be tired the next day. My body will be stiff and useless. I want to do normal things but can't. I'm tired of hearing "You can't be in that much pain." It infuriates me. Imagine what your life would be life if you woke up every day, feeling like you were engulfed in flames. Some people think this is a joke. That fibromyalgia is just something that we exaggerate. But they have no idea what this ongoing battle is like, and they never will.

All the doctors do is apologize. I understand that there is only so much they can do, but that's still not enough. Sometimes I wonder if this is God's plan so I can share my story and help the next person who is suffering like me. Struggling for so many years with no answers. It's hard to stay positive but it's a must. This is something that I have to live with for the rest of my life. As I sat and wrote this book, the pain wasn't that bad which I would call one of my good days. I was able to cook but had to sit down several times due to my back pain. Then the sciatica pain kicked in, so I had to ask for help. While rare, there are small occasions where the pain is mild, and I truly cherish those moments.

My weight goes up and down due to no consistency with exercises. The doctor said I can do 30 minutes, but I will suffer after. I feel so defeated, but I smile through the pain because I don't want anyone feeling sorry for me.

Being the mother of a small child can get hard when she wants to do things like go to the playground, but I push through for her and suffer that night and all of the next day. We do fun stuff in the house also. I do have days when we can dance around the house, laughing and having so much fun. But once I settle down all hell breaks loose and it will be bad days for a long time. But that's the sacrifice I make for my baby girl. Once again I lay in bed wondering why me God? When people say they are in pain you have to believe them. Everyone deals with pain differently. Fibromyalgia is a long term disease with no cure. The cause of fibromyalgia is unknown, and it is believed to involve a combination of genetic factors. The pain appears to result from processes in the central nervous system and the condition is referred to as central sensitization syndrome. We are given antidepressants, anti-seizure medication, opioids and physical therapy. But most of these things don't work. Physical therapy is more pain to deal with especially for me because of my back issues.

I've been denied disability on more than one occasion. They assume that I can work. But how in the hell can I? They are assuming just like everyone else. If I could work, I would! I used to be a CNA and I loved it. But my back pain and body pain caused me to stop. I couldn't take it, I tried to stay because I love working and helping people. I tried retail also but that didn't work out either due to my pain. Even my doctors told me I'm not able to work which hurt. I hate it but I understand. I will find other things to do. I thought about network marketing but it's not for me. I keep telling myself that things will get better.

With my back also getting worse, I decided to see a specialist and get their opinion. After a few MRIs and X-rays we decided that I should get a spinal fusion. The doctor told me that my lower back was pretty much bone on bone and will get worse by the day. So my husband and I talked about it and decided that this would be the best option. the doctor claimed that I would get 80% relief and that made me happy. I've been dealing with back pain along with fibromyalgia for years.

May 1, 2018 was the day of the surgery, but before I could have the procedure, I had to get a medical clearance. The doctor explained how I would be in the hospital for about 2 weeks, which I wasn't prepared for because I was previously told something different.

19

After my surgery, I woke up 6 hours later in so much pain all I could do was cry. My face was swollen, my right leg was numb, and the pain was unbearable. Seventeen days later, I'm finally home, but still in pain. I kept saying to myself "I hope this gets better." Unfortunately there was no relief. The decision to do the surgery was a huge regret, and I ended up having more issues than I did before. I went from doctor to doctor for more help and still got nothing . So a year later, here I am, and my leg is still numb.

Now they say I have arthritis in my right knee which I didn't have before the surgery. Confused and angry, I still take it all day bay day. The pain in my back and down my leg was getting ridiculous, and now I'm stuck with pain no one can explain once again. My fibromyalgia flare ups are worse now. I'm getting flare ups that are lasting for days at a time. I'm getting less sleep due to this pain. The more issues that arise, the more depressed I get. I cry in the shower and it got to the point where I didn't want to go anywhere, not even to the doctors. I made all types of excuses. It was hard being around people who were filled with joy, carrying on with their everyday lives happy and carefree. But I would put my big girl panties on and that smile of mine and keep it moving. I hated that I had to use a back brace and a walker. Using the wheelchair only if we go to the mall or places similar. It's very depressing to be my age and have to use those things. I want to go out and do normal things without feeling like my body is on fire. But I have to stay positive even though some days I just want to ball up in my bed and cry.

Even when I have a good day I can't do too much because I will pay for it the next day or the pain will last for days. People say that I'm so strong but at times I don't know how to feel. When dealing with fibromyalgia, you have to try to be strong because it's the life you live. They say God won't give you more than you can handle. I guess I'm handling things pretty good. I don't even know how I managed to write all this, because my hands kept swelling up. But I kept pushing. Nobody wants to look sick, so of course I won't always look sick.

I pray a lot and I have to try and stay positive. Never give up no matter what how hard it gets. This too shall pass. Whatever it is that you wat to do in life, you just have to find other ways to do it. Listen to your body when you feel like you need to rest please do so. Dealing with fibromyalgia, you never know what you will get each day. My feet swell up from time to time which hurt like hell. I get random breakouts too. If you don't have a good support group this can get hard on you. But it can also be hard on your family. I know it's hard on my family, but they will continue to stay positive right along with me. My husband is the absolute best! On my restless nights he stays up with me. We will watch tv or sometimes he rubs my back or legs to help me relax so I can go to sleep. I really appreciate everything he does to help me get some relief.

My best friend Terri didn't understand it until she was around me when I was having a bad flare up. So now she knows it's real. See, you will have those who don't believe you can be that sick until they see it for themselves. But it's ok because they don't live in your body. My cousin Jada understands completely because she too has fibromyalgia. Some family members think they get it, but don't completely understand. For that, I'm thankful for my support team. I want to one day speak to people in my area that are dealing with chronic pain just like me. Maybe we can come together and teach people how to understand what we go through. This is also why I wrote this book. I want to find a doctor who doesn't want to just throw me pills all the time. Let's find some holistic stuff and not pills. I also wish doctors would listen, and stop using their position to assume they know everything. We are the ones suffering every day, not them. I don't want to be stuck on pills for the rest of my life, which is why I expressed interest in going the holistic route. These medications have effects that do harm to the body as we age, and I don't want any more issues than I already have. I'm hoping that trying a plant based diet can be beneficial in giving my body what it needs to heal.

Can you imagine your body hurting from head to toe? No you can't!! But this is my life! This isn't for the weak, but it can break you. I will say, if you feel like you need to cry then let it out. Don't keep it in like I did and now I'm dealing with depression. I kept telling myself it couldn't be me. That I was okay, but it was a lie. Holding it all in was nightmare, and eventually I gave in emotionally and broke down. I'm always tired. Fatigue is bad with fibromyalgia. The more rest you get is good. But it's hard to sleep when my legs hurt and feel like someone is sticking pins in them. I struggled to write this book, but I'm determined to get my story out.

So let's talk about disability. Why do these people feel that we can work in our condition? They are quick to deny us, but they have no idea of what we deal with every day. And I'm sure they don't care. They make you feel bad, and claim that you can do simple, menial jobs which isn't true. One judge had the nerve to tell me if I can move my arms and legs I can work. That pissed me off! I wanted to scream! But again, she doesn't understand what I go through. Yes I can move my arms and legs, but pain comes with it. They don't care, because their lives are normal. They aren't me. I wish they could be in my shoes for just one day. Then I know for sure their mentality would change. My struggles with employment and disability benefits is why I hate to hear a person complain about their job, knowing I can't work. I go to the doctors more than anything. So I guess that's my job.

I've learned so much living this life of pain. Don't judge anyone because you never know what they are going through. You have to be very optimistic when it comes to living with chronic pain. It's no joke. You learn how to smile when u want to cry. So now on my real bad days I cry it out and put some music on to try and get my mind off the pain. They say that it's no cure for fibromyalgia, but I pray one day they find something. Soon I will need to get a handicap sticker for my husband's truck because now he drops me off in the front of the store, so I don't have to walk far. If I walk too long or stand too long, my body will start to burn. Walking in the grocery store is rough since I have to hold on to the cart and pray I make it until we are done. Like I said before, with fibromyalgia you don't know what will happen. I get all types of pain everywhere. It can go from my feet on up. Like stick pins.

I got married in July of 2018. It was such an amazing day for me. Even though I had to take meds just to walk down the aisle. I also had on a back brace. I was smiling from ear to ear but crying inside. When we got home I crashed. I was in so much pain and so exhausted I just took my dress off and was out for hours. My husband understood. That day was very special to me, so I pushed through for the both of us. Chronic pain is no fun. People told me that I looked like I had gained weight on my wedding day. All I could do was laugh because it wasn't fat, I was swollen from a flare up. I even had to wear sneakers on my wedding day because of my back and legs. But even in sneakers, I slayed on my wedding day and fibromyalgia wouldn't stop my shine! I wish my mom could've been there to witness my big day, but I know she is resting in heaven smiling down on me. I believe that the rain we had that day were her tears of joy. I'm sure she's proud of the woman I've become. I promised her I would find more natural things to help me and I'm dedicated to keeping that promise.

Sometimes I lay on the couch wondering what if? I go from heating pad to ice packs . I have to switch it up at times. I've tried all the pain creams, but they only help if I'm having a low pain day and that's not often. The last time I cooked my family a big dinner, boy did I pay for it! Even though I took my time and sat down between preparation. That pain hit my body so fast all I could do was cry. But that's what happens when people with chronic pain try to have a normal day like everyone else.

Another day, I rode with my husband to the store. I just wanted to get some fresh air. I ended up on the couch when we returned home, wishing I hadn't. I had pillows all under me and an ice pack on my hip. My daughter wanted her hair braided so I had to push through and attend to my motherly duties, but again, the pain came after. One day I want to be able to travel, but not until I can get this pain under control. I wake up with headaches, then off to the pharmacy I go to get more meds. The pharmacist told me the meds won't help with chronic pain if taken with a low dosage. But this is what the doctor put me on so what can I do? I'll come home, eat lunch, then spend the rest of my time resting. Finally I'll fall asleep for a few hours.

The doctor always says if I'm tired try to take a nap but then I'm up all night. So I do what I can. Most nights I'm up in pain anyway. Now I have to deal with this concerning fluid in my ankle. My ankle swells everyday now. But like other recent issues, I suspect that it's due to my horrible surgery. For years it's been my lower back that hurt but now it's my entire back. These doctors complain about there are so many people addicted to narcotics, but they are the ones prescribing and having people take them 3-4 times a day. I can't take them that much. I would be sleeping all day long, and I can't function like that. I feel like they just want us high out of our minds, and wandering around in a zombified state. But either way the meds don't take the pain away, so they can prescribe all they want.

Every day I pray for a cure! One day I woke up around 9 am with throbbing pain in my ankle. I had my morning coffee and took my meds. Same crap, different day. I read my affirmations and that helped relax my mind. I did let my husband know about the new issues with my ankle because the fluid was just sitting. I ended up in bed all day with a heating pad. Living with chronic pain I never know what type of day I'm going to have, but I thank God for waking me up each day. I have to embrace my good days. Chronic pain is like the aches and exhaustion you get with the flu. Or how you feel after an intense workout but worse. Having flares that make you feel like you've been hit by a car. Yet chronic pain is usually invisible. This means that most people don't understand how someone can be in pain all the time. Want to imagine what fibromyalgia feels like? First catch the flu, and then get a bad sunburn all over. Stay awake for 36 hours straight. You'll get IBS and some swelling. Don't even get me started on the fatigue. The pain can go from 0-100 quick. It's very unpredictable.

One day you feel good then the next day you feel like crap. Or you might not even be able to get out of bed. I am a very strong woman. Everything that comes my way in life I've dealt with head on. I've cried plenty of nights, but I also picked myself back up . I've grown from the things that were meant to break me and I'm getting stronger by the day. My faith is #1. Without my faith this thing called fibromyalgia would break me every single day. But I'm determined to one day be able to have women come together and talk about the things we go through. We need to educate people to rid them of their ignorance.

Fibromyalgia not only affects our body with lots of pain, but it also affects our emotions. It makes us lonely, moody, emotional, sad, depressed, angry and irritable. You just never know. I wake up tired. I go to sleep tired. I wake up in pain. I go to sleep in pain. My weight goes up and down thanks to the medication.

I always say you have to be strong to deal with chronic pain. I have other issues too. Chronic pain will have you down for days. But people need to understand my body is different from yours so I can't just get up and go because you can. But I damn sure wish I could. I will keep trying to live my best life with fibromyalgia. I have plans to do so much more. So world here I come, pain and all!

I want to thank everyone who's been right by my side each step of the way. Thanks for being my support team. Now that I think about I probably had this when I was in my 20s . They say stress can cause it. Ex: car accident, physical abuse etc. and I've had a few stressful issues in my life that were very bad. I'm so blessed to be in a better place in my life and that's why I try my best not to complain. I can handle all that comes my way. I will take it as it comes and move on. I pray my kids will never endure this pain. I would lose it if my kids had to endure this nightmare. Keep your kids as healthy as possible. Give them plenty of vitamins. Fibromyalgia is an illness that causes widespread destruction to your body with lots of pain, and other issues may follow. I feel like even though many will read this, some still won't get it unless they have fibromyalgia. My pain has taught me to appreciate everything that doesn't hurt. Just because you see me smiling or even see me out and about trying to live a normal life doesn't mean my pain is gone. So please don't judge me when you haven't walked in my shoes!

When you suffer from this illness, sometimes your body will twitch. Some foods can trigger fibromyalgia flare ups like red meat, gluten and eggs. Stay warm because the cold months will beat you up if you don't. The pain associated with fibromyalgia tends to fluctuate and worsen. Some natural remedies for fibromyalgia are 5-htp for the brain chemical serotonin. Fibromyalgia is not generally considered a progressive disorder but in some cases like mine it does get worse over time. Exercise can help maintain bone mass improve balance reduce stress and increase strength. Stress can trigger a flare up fast. Some medication can make you gain weight . In 2012 social security explained how fibromyalgia should be found as a medically determinable impairment, even though they still deny people benefits on a regular basis.

As painful as this is, having fibromyalgia will make you stronger than you thought you ever thought you could be. This pain is an everyday, struggle but I don't want it to take over my life. I know it's been hard for my husband to see me in so much pain and to take me to the hospital constantly. But we are strong and won't give up. He loves me and I admire his will the remain strong for me. It was truly a struggle trying to write this book. Hands swollen, feel swollen but I was determined to let people know this pain is real. It's a daily struggle just to get out of bed but I press on. Especially having a young child. I don't want anybody to feel sorry for me because I will stay smiling no matter what. Yes it's rough, but I have a family that needs me. Like I said before this pain is not for the weak. I miss working as a CNA but hey life goes on. No matter how much I tell people about this pain they will never truly understand. All we can do is keep trying to educate them. It's a fight daily but I pray one day more people will understand what we go through instead of assuming it's not that bad. Even though it's hard on my family at times, I know I can always count on them. Some understand and some don't want to understand and it's fine. But it's never okay to be negative about something you don't understand. My new outlook on life is to take it as is and keep moving.

I'm happy to say that I finally did it! I told my story!

The Pain Within Me

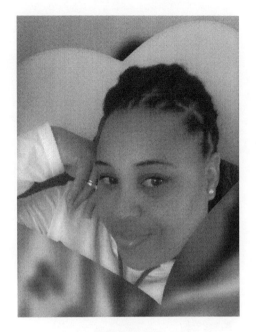

About Me

My name is Lawawn Dunbar. I'm a 46-year-old wife, mother, sister and a very good friend to others. I have 3 amazing kids, and 3 beautiful grandchildren.
I graduated from high school in 1990 and from there I went on to become a certified CNA. I love reading and doing crossword puzzles. I'm a big hearted person who would help anyone if I could.
I wrote this book to let the world know that fibromyalgia is real. I feel if more people understood it, that would make life easier on all those who suffer with this disease.

37

Resources

Fibromyalgia support group database by state - https://fibroandpain.org/support-groups

Fibromyalgia support community- https://fibroandpain.org/fibromyalgia-support-community-2

Leading organizations and charities- https://www.verywellhealth.com/leading-fibromyalgia-charities-and-organizations-4145779

Donate to the National Fibromyalgia Association- https://www.verywellhealth.com/leading-fibromyalgia-charities-and-organizations-4145779

Donate to the Fibromyalgia treatment center- https://www.verywellhealth.com/leading-fibromyalgia-charities-and-organizations-4145779

The Pain Within Me

Thanks for reading!

Made in the USA
Las Vegas, NV
31 March 2022

46644662R00025